Ketogenic Diet

The Ultimate guide for beginners

By Holly Barnes

Blueleo Media

Table of Contents

Introduction

First impressions can last a lifetime. But I probably don't need to tell you that; people might already have pigeon-holed you because of their first impression of you.

People at your workplace might have pigeon-holed you. Seeing you hard at work in your cubbyhole on your first day of work, they might have pegged you as being someone who doesn't know how to have a good time. And that first impression might have been reinforced by the fact that they've seen you plugging away in that corner every day since, especially if they've seen you with your hair down, so everyone would probably think you're no fun at all.

You might be completely misunderstood.

Just like the Ketogenic Diet.

The Ketogenic (or Keto) Diet was developed in the 1920's as a cure for epilepsy, yet people have only recently started accepting the fact that it's also great diet for weight loss. Yes, that's right. The Keto Diet was completely misunderstood for ninety years.

Can you imagine that? I mean, how would you feel if you'd slaved away in your corner cubbyhole for ninety years, with everyone thinking you're only good for epilepsy?

People definitely thought Mr. Keto was no fun at all.

But now, finally, people are getting the chance to see Mr. Keto with his hair down, and people are starting to realize how great the Keto Diet is for losing weight.

Why did it take so long for the medical establishment to find out how great the Keto Diet is for losing weight?

Mainly because, when people first heard about the diet, it seemed too good to be true. How could you possibly lose weight on a diet consisting of 75% fat? So, not only did everyone think Mr. Keto was no fun, they also thought he was off his rocker, like the guy in your office who dyes his hair purple (unless everyone in your workplace has purple hair, in which case they'd think the brunette was nuts).

But thankfully, recent research has demonstrated the Keto Diet's amazing ability to not only shed pounds, but keep them off. And yet Keto dieters eat an amazing variety of foods that normally aren't eaten by people concerned with losing weight.

How is this possible?

Because, you see, Mr. Keto had a trick up his sleeve, a mischievous trick to fool your body into shedding pounds by forcing it to burn up its stored fat.

You probably already know from long experience how hard it is to burn off those layers of stored fat. But Mr. Keto's diet does it, by lowering your intake of carbohydrates drastically.

You might be one of the many dieters who've tried to basically starve themselves to burn off that fat. Fasting is indeed a good way to induce the body to burn fat, because the body needs to burn something to generate the energy it needs, and fasting denies the body its normal energy source.

But fasting, unfortunately often leads to over-eating afterward. And fasting is tough to do. Hes, we do recommend an occasional fast, but fasting alone is seldom enough for losing a significant amount of weight, because it can only be used sporadically.

But Mr. Keto has developed a trick for making the body think it's fasting. During a fast, the body starts going into a state of ketosis, which means it starts to burn fat instead of carbohydrates to produce the energy it needs. The Keto Diet duplicates that process.

A lot of dieters are used to half-starving themselves every day, but that is unnecessary with the Keto Diet. If you're hungry on the Keto Diet, you eat. So if continually half-starving yourself is your thing, well, I guess you'll have to find another weight-loss diet.

Over the course of this book, we'll provide you with more details about this amazing diet, as well as giving you a history of the diet and recommendations for implementing it. We'll also talk about the lifestyle challenges you might be facing and how they can negatively affect your ability to lose weight.

We'll also discuss the risks the diet might pose for certain people, and how to test yourself to determine whether the diet is working properly. We'll even discuss the effects you can expect to feel from the diet. And of course we'll go into detail about how this amazing diet works better than low-calorie diets. We'll even throw in plenty of solid and delicious recipes for the diet.

Over the past few years, the Keto Diet's propensity for shedding pounds have been backed up by research testimonials. And, miraculous as the diet sounds, scientists and nutritionists have finally started to climb on board with the idea of using the Keto Diet for losing weight.

So Mr. Keto is finally getting the scientific recognition he's been deserving of for nearly a century. And all is well in Mr. Keto's life, now.

Well, almost, anyway. Mr. Keto still has some work to do on changing his image, starting with a make-over on his name. Ketogenic? Are you kidding me? I mean, really! Definitely a name out of the 1920's.

Mr. Keto has to come up with something sexy, like The Have-Your-Cake-and-Eat-It Diet. Actually, come to think of it, there might be too many carbs in that name, though I suppose you could make a low-carb cake. I'll check into that and let you know.

What Is the Ketogenic Diet?

The Ketogenic Diet is a diet high in fat and low in carbohydrates, with an adequate amount of protein.

The average diet has a high, or at least medium amount of carbohydrates. When you eat a normal meal, your body converts the carbs you eat into glucose, a type of sugar. This glucose is then used as the primary energy source for your body, while most or all of the fat that you eat is stored in the body as a potential future source of energy.

However, when you greatly reduce your intake of carbs—including while you're fasting or sleeping—your body loses its normal source of energy, carbs. This signals your body to start unlocking the fat stored in the body, and your liver starts converting this fat into ketone bodies, which pour into your bloodstream to replace glucose as your body's primary source of energy. As these ketones rush in to replace the glucose, your bloodstream is said to be in a state of "ketosis."

The standard Keto Diet, originally developed to treat epilepsy patients, contains a four-to-one ratio of fat to the combined proteins and carbohydrates, with just enough protein for body growth and repair. This ratio is achieved by reducing or even eliminating high-carb foods like starchy fruits and vegetables, bread, pasta, sugar and grains, while increasing the quantity of fatty foods like nuts, cream and butter.

Eating a high proportion of fatty foods makes you feel sated, so you often wind up eating less than you would on a low-fat diet. And because you don't feel hungry all the time, your tension levels decrease and you don't develop guilt feelings from eating fatty foods.

Originally, the Keto Diet didn't discriminate in its choice of types of fat to eat. But after new research came out about fats, the Keto Diet was revised to emphasize the consumption of medium-chain triglycerides (MCTs) from foods like coconut oil, because this type of fat contains more ketones than normal fat, which is largely composed of long-chain triglycerides (LCTs).

The original Keto Diet also restricted the intake of fluids. But because this sometimes led to the production of kidney stones in patients, that restriction has been lifted by many practitioners.

Unlike many other diets, the Keto Diet can often help treat certain conditions that might make it hard for you to lose weight, like sleep disorders, gut dysbiosis, chronic fatigue and other health problems.

The Keto Diet encourages the eating of natural foods, as opposed to some of the other diets out there that push a bunch of processed powders full of artificial ingredients at you. So you can remain on the Keto Diet for the rest of your life. And it can change your life forever.

There's a certain flexibility in the diet to allow for differences in people and their needs, so the exact ratios of fats to carbs and proteins can vary slightly from person-to-person.

You could basically say that there are four basic types of Keto Diets, standard, high-protein, targeted and cyclical. The first two have been studied extensively and have been used by many people. The last two (cyclical and targeted) have not been studied extensively and are basically intended for athletes and body-builders. We don't recommend the last two diets at all for most people. Athletes and body-builders should only use them under the supervision of a person trainer, if at all.

And remember, when you're counting carbs, you need to subtract the grams of fiber from the total grams of carbs.

The four types of Keto Diets:

Standard: Low carb, moderate protein and high fat. It typically contains 75% fat, 20% protein and 5% carbs. This is the diet we recommend in this book for the vast majority of people.

High-protein: 60% fat, 35% protein, 5% carbs. We only recommend this diet in special cases where it's definitely been demonstrated that the person requires extra protein.

Cyclical: This diet involves periods of higher carb re-feeds, such as five ketogenic days followed by two high-carb days. Recommended only for athletes and body-builders under supervision of a specialist, if at all.

Targeted: This diet allows you to add carbs around work-outs. Like the cyclical, it's mainly been used by body-builders and athletes, and is somewhat lacking in research. Recommended only for athletes and body-builders under supervision of a specialist, if at all.

Keto Diet's History

In 1921, researcher Rollin Woodyatt found that the body produced three water-soluble compounds—collectively known as ketone bodies—when a person fasted or went on a low-carbohydrate diet. Because fasting had proven effective in the treatment of epilepsy, the medical establishment experimented with using the Keto Diet to treat epilepsy.

Not only did the Keto Diet prove effective in treating epilepsy, but epileptic patients could remain on the diet on a long-term basis without the obvious drawbacks and complications of fasting. So the medical establishment approved the diet for the treatment of epilepsy.

Pediatrician Mynie Peterman formulated the classic Keto Diet, and in 1925 reported that the diet had proven effective in reducing epileptic seizures in 95% of the thirty-seven patients she'd tested, with 60% of them becoming seizure-free.

The diet gained great popularity in the treatment of epilepsy in the 1920s and 1930s, until new anti-convulsive drugs were developed to treat epilepsy. The diet declined in use after than, mainly being confined to usage by the 25% of patients for whom because the anti-convulsive drugs proved to be ineffective.

In the 1960s, people began using the Keto Diet for weight loss, but for the most part, the diet continued to toil in relative obscurity. That began to change in the 1990's, with TV exposure about how the diet had cured two cases of epileptic children where pharmaceutical treatment had failed. The first case was aired in 1994 on NBC's Dateline, concerning the son of Hollywood producer Jim Abrahams. The second case was aired in 1997, in a true-to-life movie entitled *First Do No Harm,* starring Meryl Streep.

This TV exposure sparked renewed interest in the diet, and after the turn of the century, scientists began studying it for other uses besides epilepsy, including the treatment of numerous other diseases, and many of the results were favorable. But it took awhile for the scientific community to wrap its head around the idea that the diet might be good for losing weight, so the evidence has only started to pour out recently. But even so, studies have shown that low-carbohydrate diets do indeed result in more weight loss than balanced diets. The public is ahead of the researchers now, as the diet has exploded in popularity, and the results are speaking for themselves.

Tips for Getting Started

Tip #1: Stick to 30-100 grams of net carbs per day.

By "net carbs," we mean the total carbohydrate intake minus the amount of fiber. Yes, fiber is a type of carb. But fiber passes through the digestive system without being digested or used, so you don't need to count it toward your total carbs. So, just subtract the grams of fiber from the total grams of carbs.

This tip allows you to add more high-fiber vegetables to your diet without throwing off your ratio of fats to carbs and protein. It also allows you to feel fuller at the table while eating fewer calories. Not all vegetables are labeled for fiber content, but you get get that info online at various nutrition-counting sites like SELF Nutrition Data.

Tip#2: Determine a calorie level that's right for you.

Not everyone has the same rate of metabolism or the same nutritional needs, so a little tinkering is usually necessary until you get things right.

Basically, you're shooting for just enough calories to satisfy your hunger and keep your energy levels up. Too few calories will leave you feeling tired, and too many will prevent you from losing as much weight.

But remember that anytime you make a significant change in your diet, it will throw your system off a bit at first, so you'll probably need to tinker with your calorie levels at first, until your body adapts to the changes.

Tip #3: Monitor any side effects you might experience during the early stages of the diet.

People react differently to changes in diet. Symptoms might include dizziness, fatigue, quickening heart rate and shortness of breath. If any of these symptoms occur, it's probably a good idea to avoid strenuous activity, though light exercise is probably fine and might well help alleviate the symptoms. If these symptoms seem serious or if they persist for more than a few days, it's probably a good idea to talk to your doctor.

Monitoring side effects is especially important for diabetics and other people with insulin problems who might be prone to ketoacidosis, a dangerous condition.

Tip #4: Test your ketone levels and compare the results to your meal choices.

The main idea behind this diet is to raise the level of ketones in your bloodstream, ensuring that you're entering ketosis and burning fat instead of glucose. To keep track of this, you should test your ketone levels daily and compare them to what you ate that day. This will give you graphic evidence of what's going on in your body so that you can make the proper choices to regulate your diet. In particular, it will help in determining the ideal level of carbs you should be eating.

Determining Your Ketone Levels

Here are four methods for determining your ketone levels:

#1. Judging from Symptoms of Ketosis

This doesn't cost money, but it isn't as reliable as the other methods, nor does it give you the exact levels of ketones. The normal symptoms that your body is entering ketosis can vary from person-to-person, but here are the most common:

(1). Increased urination.

(2). Dry mouth and increased thirst. It's okay to counter this by drinking more water. You can also add salt to your diet, unless salt causes you issues or you have problems with high blood pressure.

(3). Acetone breath. Acetone is a ketone that can be excreted through the breath; it has a fruity smell. This symptom is normally temporary.

(4). Increased energy. You might experience a temporary decline in energy when you first go onto the diet as your body adjusts to the change. But oftentimes, once your body makes the adjustment to the diet and enters ketosis, you'll experience higher levels of energy.

(5) Reduced hunger. Because fat is a steadier and more reliable source of energy than glucose, once you start entering ketosis, you're apt to experience fewer and milder hunger pangs.

#2. Urine Strips

Urine strips are the easiest and cheapest way to definitely determine whether you've entered ketosis, though you won't know the exact ketone levels. You can buy these strips online or from any drug store. The instructions can vary from brand to brand, but normally you just pee in a cup and dip the strip into it for about fifteen seconds. The strip will turn a different color if you're in ketosis, as per the instuctions.

One problem with urine strips is that they only are completely reliable for at most a few weeks, because your body then becomes more efficient at reabsorbing ketones from urine, so you won't be losing as many ketones to your urine. So you should make sure you use the urine strips daily from the beginning of your diet and continue using them after you start getting positive results. And then, if you start getting negative results, you can switch to a different method for monitoring your ketone level.

#3. Breath Analyzer. These instruments determine ketosis levels from your breath. Like urine strips, they give you a color code for a general ketone level rather than an exact measurement, and they aren't always completely reliable. You can get them for about $150 online or in drug stores.

#4. Blood Ketone Meter. These babies measure ketone levels exactly and are much more reliable than the other three choices. They're similar to the test diabetics use for testing their blood sugar. You prick the side of your finger to get a drop of blood and then put the drop on a strip for a machine to measure. It's usually an easy and straightforward process. Just follow the instructions and dispose of the needles properly. These meters cost about $100 and include several strips.

Analyzing Your Ketone Levels

Ketone levels can be divided into four ranges:

(1) Under 0.5 mmol/L. This is below the ketosis line, so you're burning little or no fat. You should cut down on your carb intake, and possibly your protein intake as well.

(2) From 0.5 to 1.5 mmol/L. This is a good reading for beginners on the diet, indicating a gradual transitional into a ketosis state. It means you're burning fat at a decent rate. You could continue to gradually reduce your carbs further to optimize your fat-burning.

(3) From 1.5 to 3 mmol/L. This is the optimal range to shoot for, though it isn't necessary that you reach it in order to lose weight.

(4) Readings higher than 3 mmol/L. Readings over 3 mmol/L not only don't offer any more benefit than the previous range, but can be quite dangerous. Readings this high often stem from someone who has type 1 diabetes, and these people should have been under doctor's advisement before starting the Keto Diet. If symptoms like nausea, vomiting, abdominal pain and confusion occur, it probably means you have ketoacidosis, a condition that is quite dangerous and is a medical emergency.

Twenty Things You Shouldn't Do on this Diet

Adjusting to any new diet can be tough, and sometimes people make it even harder by making mistakes. Here are twenty common mistakes people make on the Keto Diet.

1. Not Transitioning Slowly Enough to the Diet. Too many people want to jump right in and make big changes so they can lose a lot of weight in a hurry. This can produce a lot of stress on your body and your emotions. For one thing, it can cause bladder issues, making you go to the bathroom frequently. You should transition slowly to this diet, gradually increasing your fat intake and lowering you carb and protein intakes over the first two or three weeks until you arrive at the proper ratios. This will allow your body the time it needs to make a smooth transition to the ketosis state.

2. Obsessing about Your Weight. Your weight can vary quite a bit by the amount of water you drink at a particular time, so weighing yourself isn't an effective

way to determine your progress. For the first few weeks of the program, the most important thing is for your body to make a smooth adjustment to the process of burning fat; losing weight is secondary at this point. If you obsess about it you're liable to overdo things, which can harm your body or burn yourself out on the diet. Obsessing leads to added stress and eventual disappointment. This diet is all about making it through the long haul; endurance races favor the tortoise over the hare.

3. Obsessing about Your Ketone Levels. Though it's a good idea to keep track of your levels, worrying about them only makes things worse, possibly leading to depression. For the first few weeks, maintaining a positive state of mind is critical for your long-term success. On this diet, you want your body to feel good during the transition period, so the less stress and disappointment you feel, the better you'll make it through the transition. If you make it through the transition period with a positive attitude, you'll soon start burning layers of fat off.

4. Eating the Wrong Fats. Avoid oils made from vegetables or seeds. Use saturated fats like animal fats,

coconut oil and butter. Monounsaturated fats like olive oil are also good. Nuts are another good food.

5. Focusing Solely on Eliminating Carbs. Though cutting back on carbs is important, completely eliminating them is probably not be a good idea. Some people need more carbs than others, and certain carbs—like non-starchy vegetables—are quite good for the body, especially those that are high in fiber. Moderation and variety in the diet can be beneficial not only to your body but for your emotional satisfaction and well-being.

6. Overeating Protein. Though protein is absolutely essential for maintaining your organs and muscles, eating too much can hinder or even prevent your body from entering ketosis, because excess protein can be converted into glucose. So remember to monitor your protein intake closely, eating neither too little nor too much of it.

7. Not Eating Sufficient Amounts of Fat. It's tough for most dieters to get used to the idea of eating a lot of fat, but you need to do it for this diet to work. So

just enjoy all the yummy fat without feeling guilty about it.

8. Overeating Processed Foods. The Keto Diet emphasizes eating natural foods. Yes, natural foods take longer to prepare, but if you plan your meals ahead of time and make sure you have the ingredients handy, it saves you quite a bit of time in running to the store. Occasionally eating a little processed is okay for a little variety, but it isn't real food.

9. Not Getting Sufficient Salt, Minerals and Vitamins. Sometimes, people on this diet are so concerned about getting the proper proportions of fat, protein and carbs that they forget about basic nutrients. And yes, a little salt is good for the body. Too much salt can cause inflammation in a person who eats too many unnatural foods, but eating a couple teaspoons a day on a natural diet is fine.

10. Consuming Too Much Alcohol. Drinking alcohol not only adds unnecessary carbs and bad sugars to your diet, but can also interfere with your body's ability to remain in ketosis. While it's okay to

occasionally indulge a little, it's best to keep alcohol to a minimum.

11. Eating on Too Rigid of a Schedule. While a family meal schedule can sometimes be necessary in our hectic modern lives, it's important on this diet to listen to the needs of your body. Whenever possible, if you're hungry, eat. If you aren't, don't. The body is a lot wiser than we give it credit for, and trying to impose your own schedule upon it can throw off your body's rhythms.

12. Not Committing Yourself Fully to the Diet. Maintaining the proper proportions of fat to carbs is important. If you continually slack off and allow yourself to indulge in extra carbs, you can wind up with a high-fat, high-carb diet, which can not only terminate your ketosis and quickly add pounds, but can be harmful to your health.

13. Obsessing about Your Cholesterol Levels. Many people believe that cholesterol is bad, while in fact it's essential for your body. The doctor who originally came up with the idea that cholesterol leads

to heart disease eventually rejected the idea after examining the research on the subject.

14. Believing the Keto Diet Is a Quick Fix. The diet isn't a quick fix that will cure whatever ails you and instantly start burning off a lot of fat. Forget all the commercials about miracle diets that burn x number of pounds in x number of days. Not only are those stories questionable, but many of those testimonials are from people who eventually put a lot of those pounds back on.

15. Not Being Prepared for the Onset of Ketosis. Some people get the "Keto flu" when they first enter ketosis. Typical symptoms are any or all of the following: headache, stomach ache, nausea, fatigue, sleepiness and lack of mental clarity. Symptoms can last from a day to a week. You can usually avoid this by transitioning to the new diet over a period of two or three weeks. Drinking lots of water helps prevent the keto flu, mainly because entering ketosis can cause you to urinate more frequently. You can also lose electrolytes like sodium, magnesium and potassium in your urine, so make sure you replace those electrolytes. Transitioning slowly to the new diet can also help you

avoid withdrawal symptoms stemming from lowering your intake of carbs and sugar.

16. Comparing Your Progress to Others'. This is a trap that's hard to avoid falling into. People's bodies are different, so your progress has nothing to do with the progress of anyone else. Don't let yourself get discouraged if you aren't progressing as rapidly as someone else, because this discouragement can zap your will to continue the diet.

17. Allowing Setbacks in Your Progress to Impede Further Progress. Hey, we all blow it sometime, falling prey to temptation. Shake it off and accept the fact that you aren't perfect. Is anyone? Just dust yourself off and get back on track.

18. Trying to Go It Alone. While some people succeed in this diet going Lone Ranger, it's much easier to do with a good support system in place. If your family nags you about the diet, it makes it harder to go through the process. If they do nag, you'll probably either need to shut them up or shut them off and find some other support system. Online support groups are

available and can often make a great deal of difference in helping you stick with the diet.

19. Not Fasting at All. Occasionally, your body needs a break from eating. Sometimes your body will drop hints that it needs a break; maybe you'll lose your appetite or get sick, which can be signs you need to fast a day or two. Fasting can also aid in establishing or re-establishing a ketosis state.

20. Not Getting Proper Exercise. Health expert unanimously agree that proper exercise is beneficial for your body. This doesn't necessarily mean running a marathon or taking up weight-lifting. Exercise programs should be entered gradually; extremes should be avoided. A couple short, relaxed walks every day might be all the exercise you need at the beginning. Then you can gradually start working your way to a more complete regimen.

Challenges in Your Lifestyle

Most of us are involved in a hectic modern lifestyle. Unfortunately, this lifestyle can lend itself to two major problems that often lead to overeating: stress and sleep deprivation. Though they're related, we'll deal with them one at a time.

Stress

Stress—particularly if it's chronic—can not only sabotage your efforts to lose weight, but can also lead you to gain weight.

When you're stressed, it can provoke your body to enter into the fear response state (also called the flight-or-fight response), which is a natural process the body goes into when you're in a dangerous situation that requires immediate action, like facing a bear. In this situation, you need an immediate source of energy to either flee the bear or fight it.

So, your body releases adrenaline into the blood stream and increases the flow of oxygen and glucose to the brain, while also suppressing non-emergency functions like digestion. Once the danger passes, your bodily responses return to normal.

But in today's society, stress is the most common trigger of the fear response state, and stress isn't something you can fight or run away from. All too often, stress (unlike the bear) doesn't go away. Stress can become chronic, leaving you in a permanent or semi-permanent state of low-grade fear. So your body pumps out adrenaline throughout the day and suppresses your digestive functions, while also overworking your heart.

Under stress, the body—thinking it's in survival mode—releases the hormone cortisol, which makes you feel hungry. The body does this because it assumes you're going to be burning calories in order to fight or flee from the bear, and therefore burn a lot of calories that will need to be replaced. So your body starts to crave carbohydrates, because carbs provide you with energy-producing glucose. In short, your body has been tricked into thinking you need to eat, so you eat.

And gain weight.

There are numerous relaxation techniques for dealing with stress (deep breathing exercises, meditation, relaxing exercises, massage, etc.) that might help you, but they're beyond the scope of this book.

Sleep Deprivation

The busy lifestyle that produces stress can also cause sleep deprivation. In fact, stress itself can cause sleep deprivation. A lot of people suffer from stress and/or sleep deprivation without even knowing it. They might just think they're tired just from work, when in fact they aren't getting enough deep, restful sleep. They might even reach a point where they're so used to being sleep-deprived that it begins to feel normal to them.

Lack of sleep decreases the body's production of leptin, a hormone that makes you feel sated, while also triggering the production of ghrelin, a hormone that makes you feel hungry. This double whammy makes you feel hungry, even if you've eaten recently.

There are numerous causes of sleep deprivation. Among them are things that prevent you from winding down before bedtime, like watching the news—which is full of violence—or watching action or horror movies. There are numerous techniques for treating sleep deprivation, though the most common—sleeping pills—is a dangerous treatment that is only meant to be used sporadically.

But the treatments for sleep deprivation are beyond the scope of this book. There are plenty of websites devoted to dealing with stress and sleep deprivation.

Maintaining Your Good Work

Starting a weight program is largely about keeping a positive mindset and not letting setbacks discourage you. Sure, determination factors into the equation, but for some people, the real time for determination is after you've successfully started losing weight.

Yes, you heard that right. Sometimes, maintaining your good work can be harder than getting your initial success.

As they say, nothing fails like success.

If you're patting your back because you've lost ten or fifty pounds and you're starting to look good, there's a danger that you're going to relax and start sloughing off. And once you start on that path, you're in trouble.

So here are some tips for maintaining the proper attitude:

Put before-and-after photos of yourself somewhere as a reminder both of what you've accomplished and where you don't want to return.

Reward yourself regularly for your hard work, but not by eating a chocolate bar. Treat yourself to something not related to food or drink.

Yes, you can occasionally cheat slightly on your diet, but not by eating carbs, because that will confuse your body and possibly throw you out of ketosis. You could maybe give yourself a couple days a month where you cheat slightly, maybe when someone takes you out to dinner or something.

If that doesn't work, and your determination starts wavering, maybe it's time to get away for a while, or maybe you'll need to make some other change in your routine.

Remind yourself that you feel healthier now and you feel better about yourself after getting to this point.

Some people develop their own mantra that they repeat to themselves whenever they start to stray. This can re-wire your brain to stay on the straight-and-narrow.

Starting an exercise program can help, especially if it's with friends or at a gym. The gym has the advantage of prodding yourself to look good in front of new people you meet.

The gym can also be a good place to meet people who've made healthy choices and can help advise you when you start to waver. It's important to have someone to talk to who's already been through what you're going through.

Think of other ways to distract yourself from temptations that you might run into. Maybe something easy like having sugarless gum or something in your pocket, or maybe you can play a certain song when temptation starts knocking. Get creative.

The Recipes

This is the fun chapter. All the mouth-watering recipes.

Come to think of it, maybe none of the chapters above are necessary. Why on earth would you falter on this diet if you get to eat these recipes?

Seriously, though, these recipes are broken down into four categories: Breakfast, Main Meals, Snacks and Desserts.

Each recipe provides carbohydrate and protein counts in grams per serving size. These should help you stay on course. Most of these recipes serve four people.

Feel free to substitute other ingredients if necessary to suit your needs, and of course we encourage you to share these recipes with others who might be interested in them.

Breakfast

Mushroom Omelet

Ingredients

3 eggs

7/8 oz. butter, for frying

7/8 oz. shredded cheese

1/5 onion

2 – 3 mushrooms

salt and pepper

Instructions

Crack the eggs into a mixing bowl with a pinch of salt and pepper. Whisk the eggs into a batter with a fork.

Add salt and spices.

Melt butter in a frying pan and pour in the batter when the butter has melted.

When the omelet begins to cook and get firm, but still has a little raw egg on top, sprinkle cheese, mushrooms and onion on top (optional).

Using a spatula, ease around the edges of the omelet, then fold it over in half. When it starts to turn golden brown underneath, remove the pan from the heat and slide the omelet on to a plate.

Tip!

Serve the omelet with a crispy salad.

Breakfast Tapas

Ingredients

A selection of cheese (for example mozarella, cheddar, gouda and parmesan)

A selection of cold cuts (serrano ham, proscuitto, chorizo, salami)

Cucumber, peppers, radishes, pickled cucumbers

Avocado with homemade mayonnaise and pepper

Nuts, e.g. walnuts, almonds or hazelnuts (low-carb nuts guide)

fresh basil

Instructions

Cut the cold cuts, cheese and vegetables into sticks or cubes.

Split the avocado and cut into small wedges.

Scrambled Eggs

Ingredients

3 eggs

2 oz. butter

salt and pepper

Instructions

Whisk the eggs together with some salt and pepper using a fork.

Melt the butter in a non-stick skillet over medium heat. Watch carefully—the butter shouldn't turn brown!

Pour the eggs into the skillet and stir for 1 – 2 minutes, until they are creamy and cooked just shy of how you like them. Remember that the eggs are still cooking even after you've put them on your plate.

Tip!

These fluffy eggs pair well with many low-carb favorites. Obvious choices are bacon or sausage, but other great options include salmon, avocado, cold cuts, and cheese (try cheddar, fresh mozzarella, or feta).

And, if you are really hungry (or have extra-large eggs), don't be shy. Add more butter!

Keto Morning Meatloaf

Ingredients

Ghee

6 large eggs

1lb bulk sweet Italian sausage or breakfast sausage (I used Jimmy Dean's sage blend - it comes in a tube and is pre-seasoned)

1/4 yellow onion, chopped

4oz organic cream cheese at room temperature, divided

1 cup shredded cheddar cheese

2 tbsp chopped scallion

Instructions

Preheat oven to 350 degrees F

Grease small loaf pan with some ghee.

In a large bowl, lightly beat the eggs. Add the sausage, onion, and half the cream cheese. Mix thoroughly.

Pour the meatloaf and egg mixture into the loaf pan. Add to the oven and bake, uncovered, about 30 minutes or until stiff.

Remove from oven and let sit for 5 minutes. Some fat may have risen to the top and begun to cool. You can use a spoon to lightly scrape it off (it should come right off without ruining the meatloaf top.)

Spread the remaining cream cheese over the top of the meatloaf, then top it with cheddar cheese and scallions. Add the meatloaf back to the oven.

Bake for about 5 more minutes, then switch to Broil for about 2-3 or until the cheddar cheese begins to golden and crisp.

Remove from oven, and let the meatloaf sit for at least 5 minutes before slicing and serving.

Notes

Per serving: Calories: 682 | Total Fat 56g | Protein: 38g | Carbohydrates: 5g | Fiber: 0.5g | Net Carbs: 4.5g per serving.

Low Carb Blueberry Ricotta Pancakes

Ingredients

3 large eggs

¾ cup ricotta

½ teaspoon vanilla extract

¼ cup unsweetened vanilla almond milk

1 cup almond flour

½ cup golden flaxseed meal

¼ teaspoon salt

1 teaspoon baking powder

¼-½ teaspoon stevia powder

¼ cup blueberries

Instructions

1. Preheat a skillet over medium heat. Blend together the eggs, ricotta, vanilla extract, and unsweetened almond milk.

3. Mix together the almond flour, golden flaxseed meal, salt, baking powder, and stevia in a separate bowl.

4. Slowly add the dry ingredients into the blender, and blend until a smooth batter forms.

5. For the ¼ cup of blueberries, you will need to add 2-3 blueberries per pancake. Exact number of berries you have will depend on their size, so feel free to halve them if needed.

6. Add butter to the preheated skillet. Wait for the butter to melt.

7. Pour your pancake batter into the skillet and flip when lightly browned on the outside. To get the full number of servings, use a 2 tablespoon measurement to scoop in the batter.

8. Serve with sugar free syrup, or additional berries.

Notes

This makes a total of 5 servings of Blueberry Ricotta Pancakes. Each pancake comes out to be 296.6 Calories, 22.6g Fats, 5.9g Net Carbs, and 13.4g Protein.

Crunchy Cinnamon Keto Granola {Grain-Free, Low Carb}

Ingredients

1 cup sliced almonds

1 cup unsweetened coconut flakes

1 cup diced walnuts

2 tsp cinnamon

4 packs Splenda Naturals (a stevia/erythritol blend I prefer, but you can sweeten to taste w/ your own sweetener you have on hand).

2 tbsp coconut oil, melted

Instructions

Preheat oven to 375

Line a baking sheet with parchment paper.

In a medium sized bowl, toss all ingredients together.

Spread out mixture over the baking sheet in as much of a single layer as you can.

Add to oven and bake for about 10 minutes, or until mixture begins to brown (keep an eye on it, oven times may vary).

Remove, mix again and enjoy in a bowl with cold unsweetened almond milk.

Notes

To store, add to a ziplock bag with a paper towel to absorb any moisture.

A Crunchy Fresh Keto Cereal Recipe

Ingredients:

1 package of Flaked Coconut

Ground cinnamon

Stevia (optional)

Unsweetened almond milk

2 medium-sized strawberries

Parchment paper / coconut oil

Instructions

Preheat your oven to 350 degrees.

If you have parchment paper, line a cookie sheet with it, if you don't, grease a cookie sheet with coconut oil. Or, come up with your own no-stick option.

Pour the coconut flakes onto the cookie sheet (use two if you want)

Cook in the oven for five minutes, watching the whole time.

Shuffle the flakes around and keep cooking until they're all a little tan and lightly toasted.

Take out the flakes.

Sprinkle lightly with cinnamon. If you want to use Stevia, sprinkle VERY lightly. Taste test until they're how you like them.

Throw 1/2 cup of the toasted chips into a bowl and pour the unsweetened Almond milk over them.

Slice up two strawberries for garnish and a little extra dash of freshness.

Enjoy!

Lunch

Keto Garlic Mascarpone Broccoli Alfredo Fried Pizza {Grain-Free}

Ingredients

1 tbsp garlic olive oil

1 cup shredded pizza cheese blend

1 cup shredded mozzarella cheese

1/4 cup mascarpone cheese

2 tbsp ghee

1 tbsp heavy cream

1 tsp minced garlic

1/8 tsp lemon pepper seasoning

2 pinches of salt

1/3 cup steamed, chopped broccoli heads

Shaved asiago cheese to taste

Instructions

Heat a medium non-stick pan to medium heat. Add olive oil and wait until it's hot and shimmers.

Add pizza cheese blend first, form into a circle (pizza blend is less likely to stick to the pan)

Add the mozzarella cheese on top and form into a circle.

Cook for 4-5 minutes until it gets crispy and you can easily slide a spatula under all the edges and can slide the crust onto a plate to cool.

Add mascarpone cheese, ghee, heavy cream, garlic, lemon pepper and salt to the hot pan, and cook for five minutes until bubbling.

Drizzle half the mixture over the crust.

Add the chopped, steamed broccoli to the other half.

Cook for about 1 minute until hot and bubbling.

Add the broccoli to the pizza.

Sprinkle shaved asiago cheese and extra lemon pepper seasoning over the top (optional)

Grain-Free Pesto-Mozzarella Fried Pizza {LCHF, Low Carb, Keto}

Ingredients

1 tbsp garlic infused olive oil

1.5 cups mozzarella cheese

1/3 cup tomato sauce (naturally low carb preferred, 3-4 net carbs or less)

Grated parmesan cheese (to taste)

Pizza/italian seasonings (to taste)

Toppings

1/4 cup mozzarella cheese

2 tbsp pesto

2 small mozzarella balls (sliced into four slices)

Instructions

Pre-heat your broiler to 500 degrees F.

Heat a good non-stick pan (I used ceramic) up to medium heat and add the garlic oil.

When the oil coats the pan and is shiny, add your mozzarella (it should start sizzling right away).

Use a spatula to spread the cheese evenly and round the corners, like a pizza.

Cook for about 3-5 minutes while it melts and starts to become dark around the edges.

Once all the cheese has melted and it's starting to brown, add the tomato sauce and spread around lightly with a spoon.

Cook for another minute or so.

Use a spatula and start sliding it around the edges of the pizza, and then underneath just to de-stick it from the pan, but not trying to lift it off the pan.

Once the pizza is free from the pan, tip your pan and slide your pizza on to a foil-lined pan (you can use your spatula to guide it)

Sprinkle your grated cheese and pizza seasonings.

Top with 1/4 cup mozzarella, a few dollops of pesto, and mozzarella slices

Put in the oven for about a minute or two until toppings are hot.

Let sit for about two minutes, while the cheese hardens and becomes crust-like.

Cut into fours, and enjoy!

Lemon Thyme Chicken on Rosemary Skewers

Ingredients

10 6" rosemary skewers (soaked in water for at least 1 hour)

1.5lbs chicken tenderloins (approx. 10)

A few sprigs of fresh thyme

1/2 tbsp garlic salt

1/2 tbsp lemon pepper seasoning

1/2 tbsp rosemary olive oil (or regular)

Instructions

Preheat oven to 350 degrees

Soak the rosemary skewers for at least 1 hour in water (3 hours max - you don't want the bark to come off, but if it does just slide it off).

Use a short sharp knife to widdle a point on the end of each of each stick.

Toss chicken with ingredients. Slide the leaves off the thyme sprigs and sprinkle them in.

Skewer each tenderloin with a rosemary stick.

Bake at 350 for 40 minutes.

Enjoy!

Keto Buffalo Wings

Serves 3

Ingredients

12 chicken wings

4 tablespoons butter

1/4 cup hot sauce (I'm a Frank's loyalist!)

1 clove of garlic, minced

1/4 tsp paprika

1/4 teaspoon cayenne pepper (for the non-mild version)

1/4 teaspoon salt

1 grind of fresh pepper

Instructions

While your chicken wings are baking, add your garlic and butter to a microwave-safe bowl.

Heat up the butter and garlic mixture in the microwave or on the stove (microwave is faster!)

Once melted into a clear liquid consistency, add the rest of the ingredients and mix together.

When your wings are cooked, toss them all in a bowl together until coated.

Low-Carb Tuna Cheese Melt

Ingredients

2 pieces of Oopsie bread or other low-carb bread

Tuna Fish Salad

5 1/3 tablespoons mayonnaise or sour cream

1 - 2 celery stalks

4 tablespoons dill pickles, chopped

1 can tuna in olive oil

½ teaspoon lemon juice

½ garlic clove, minced

salt and pepper, to taste

Topping

3½ oz. shredded cheese

1 pinch cayenne pepper or paprika powder

For serving

1/3 lb leafy greens

olive oil

Oopsie bread (makes 6-8)

3 eggs

4¼ oz. cream cheese

1 pinch salt

½ tablespoon ground psyllium husk powder

½ teaspoon baking powder

Instructions

Preheat the oven to 350° F (175° C).

Mix the salad ingredients well.

Place the bread slices on a baking sheet with parchment paper. Spread the tuna mix on the bread and sprinkle cheese on top.

Add some paprika powder or cayenne pepper.

Bake in oven until the cheese has turned a nice color, about 15 minutes. Serve the sandwich with some leafy greens drizzled with olive oil.

Oopsie bread

Separate the eggs, with the egg whites in one bowl and the egg yolks in another.

Whip egg whites together with salt until very stiff. You should be able to turn the bowl over without the egg whites moving.

Mix the egg yolks and the cream cheese well. If you want, add the psyllium seed husk and baking powder (this makes the Oopsie more bread-like).

Gently fold the egg whites into the egg yolk mix – try to keep the air in the egg whites.

Put 6 large or 8 smaller oopsies on a paper-lined baking tray.

Bake in the middle of the oven at 150° C (300° F) for about 25 minutes – until they turn golden.

Chicken Breast with Herb Butter

Ingredients

Fried chicken

4 chicken breasts

1 oz. butter or olive oil

salt and pepper

Herb butter

1/3 lb butter, at room temperature

1 garlic clove

½ teaspoon garlic powder

4 tablespoons chopped fresh parsley

1 teaspoon lemon juice

½ teaspoon salt

Leafy greens

½ lb leafy greens, for example baby spinach

Instructions

To make it extra simple to prepare herb butter, take the butter out of the fridge 30-60 minutes before starting (optional).

Start with the herb butter. Mix all ingredients thoroughly in a small bowl and let sit until it's time to serve.

Season the chicken with salt and pepper. Fry in butter or oil on medium heat until the filets are cooked through. Lower the temperature towards the end to avoid dry chicken filets.

Serve the chicken on a bed of leafy greens and let a generous amount of herb butter melt on top.

Pancakes with Savory Cream-Cheese Topping

Ingredients

1¼ eggs

2¼ oz. cottage cheese

¼ pinch salt

¼ tablespoon ground psyllium husk powder

butter or coconut oil, for frying

Topping

2 oz. cream cheese or ricotta cheese

½ tablespoon green pesto or red pesto

½ tablespoon olive oil

1/8 red onion, thinly sliced

sea salt

ground black pepper

Instructions

Mix cream cheese, 1 tablespoon olive oil and pesto. Set aside.

Mix eggs, cottage cheese, salt and psyllium husk powder with a hand blender into a smooth batter. Let sit for 10 minutes.

Heat a couple of tablespoons butter or olive oil in a large frying pan on medium heat. Put a few dollops of the cottage cheese batter, maximum 2 – 3 inches in diameter, in the pan and fry the pancakes for a few minutes on each side.

Serve with a generous amount of cream cheese mixture and a few red onion slices. Top with sea salt and freshly ground black pepper. Drizzle the remaining olive oil on top.

Tip!

If you don't have any pesto at home, you can add flavor to the cream cheese with other things, like finely chopped chives, fresh herbs or smoked fish roe.

Dinner

Keto Supreme Pizza Rolls {Low Carb, Grain-Free}

Ingredients

2 cups mozzarella cheese

1 tsp pizza seasoning

1/4 cup chopped red & green peppers

2 tbs chopped white onions

1/2 cup crumbled sausage (cooked)

1 small Campari tomato (or 2 grape tomatoes), sliced

1/4 cup pizza sauce (anything naturally low carb)

Instructions

Preheat oven to 400F

Line a small baking pan with parchment paper, leaving extra on the sides so you can lift it out of the baking sheet while it's still hot.

Use just a dab of olive oil to rub down the parchment (you'll thank me later).

Sprinkle your cheese into the baking sheet. It should be a single layer of cheese, but enough to fully cover the bottom without any holes. You may need to add more depending on HOW small your baking pan is.

Sprinkle 1 tsp pizza seasoning over the cheese.

Bake in the oven for about 20 minutes, or until cheese is browned.

Remove from oven, and try to gently slide a silicone spatula under the cheese. If you can fairly easily get it under all the sides and then the middle, then it's ready for the next step (if not, cook longer).

If it's ready, add sausage, green peppers, onions, red peppers, and sliced tomato.

Drizzle tomato sauce over the top.

If you desire, sprinkle a little more pizza seasoning on top.

Add back into the oven and cook for 10 more minutes.

Remove from oven.

Remove pizza from pan by lifting with the sides of the parchment paper.

One more time, use a silicone spatula gently to just make sure the pizza isn't sticking by sliding it under all the edges, and then the middle of the pizza.

Looking at your pizza in a horizontal view, slice 6 strips top to bottom. Then roll them top to bottom.

Let cool for about a minute to set, then enjoy!

Keto Swedish Meatballs {Grain-Free & Low Carb}

Ingredients

2 lbs ground meatloaf blend (or 1 lb ground beef and 1lb ground pork is fine)

1 cup shredded mild Cheddar cheese

1 large egg

1 tbsp water

1/4 cup diced onions

1/2 tsp ground nutmeg

1/4 tsp allspice

4 tbsp salted butter

1.5 cups chicken broth

1.5 cups heavy (whipping) cream

1 tbsp Dijon mustard

1 tbsp Worcestershire sauce

Instructions

Preheat oven to 400 degrees F and preheat a slow cooker to low.

Line a large baking pan with parchment paper

In a large bowl, combine ground meat, cheddar cheese, egg, onion, water, nutmeg and allspice.

Roll the mixture into 1.5 inch meatballs and arrange them on the lined baking pan (may require two depending on how large your pan is -- makes about 24 meatballs)

Bake for about 20 minutes or until a thermometer reads 140 degrees F.

Meanwhile, in a small skillet, heat the butter, chicken broth, and heavy cream over medium heat.

Once it begins to simmer, reduce the heat to low and let continue simmering for about 20 minutes until it reduces in half (stir frequently, especially toward the end).

Stir in the mustard and Worcestershire sauce.

Pour the sauce into a slow cooker and add the meatballs when they're ready.

Cook on low for about 2 hours so the meatballs can marinate.

Stir every half hour or so, covering all the meatballs, and don't cook in the slow cooker longer than two hours, or the sauce may start to separate.

Notes

That last instruction is key. If you don't mix and cook too long, the cream in the sauce will begin to separate (yep, I cooked it for 4 hours once and it still tasted fine but was much less pleasant to look at after 4 hours! Live and learn!)

MACROS: Calories 773 // Fat 50g // Protein 74g // Cholesterol 347mg // Carbs 3g // Fiber 0g // Net Carbs 3g

Roasted Red Pepper and Garlic Stuffed Mozzarella Chicken

Ingredients

2 tbsp extra virgin olive oil (bonus if you have garlic-infused olive oil)

2 boneless, skinless free-range chicken breasts

10 fresh basil leaves

8 small herb marinated mozzarella balls (like you find in the deli section)

6 cloves of garlic

1 roasted pepper, sliced in half the long way

1 tbsp all-purpose chicken seasoning (or your favorite seasoning for chicken)

garlic salt

freshly ground pepper

1 tbsp chopped fresh oregano (or 1 tbsp italian seasoning)

Instructions

Preheat oven to 400 degrees F

Pound slightly and then butterfly the chicken breasts

Place fresh basil in each of the breasts, then top with 4 mozzarella balls each, and squeeze garlic cloves between them.

Top with 1/2 of red pepper on top of the mozzarella.

Drizzle the marinated oil from the mozzarella over the breasts if you like, otherwise drizzle with olive oil / garlic olive oil.

Sprinkle seasoning, a decent dose of garlic salt and ground pepper over breasts.

The sprinkle chopped oregano over the whole thing.

Place in a glass baking dish, or on a baking pan with parchment paper.

Bake uncovered for 40 minutes or until internal temp reaches 180 degrees F.

Notes

If you can't find the mini mozzarella balls that are marinated in oil and herbs in your fresh deli section or olive bar, feel free to use a regular ball of mozzarella cut into 4 slices.

Spicy Sausage & Cabbage Skillet Melt

Ingredients

4 links spicy Italian chicken sausages

1 ½ cups green cabbage, shredded

1 ½ cups purple cabbage, shredded

½ cup diced onion

2 Tbsp. coconut oil

2 slices (1 ounce each) Colby Jack cheese

2 Tbsp. fresh cilantro, chopped

Instructions

1. Remove casings from sausages and rough chop. Chop onion and shred cabbage if not using pre-shredded cabbage.

2. Melt coconut oil in a large skillet and add onion and cabbage. Cook over medium-high heat until the vegetables begin to become tender, about 8 minutes.

3. Add sausage, stirring to mix it into the cabbage and onions. Cook 8 minutes more.

4. Add the cheese on top and cover the skillet.

5. Turn off the heat and wait 5 minutes while the cheese melts into the cabbage and vegetables.

6. Remove the lid from the skillet and stir. Top with cilantro and serve immediately right from the skillet.

This makes a total of 4 servings Spicy Sausage & Cabbage Skillet Melt. Each serving comes out to be 231 Calories, 14.62g Fats, 3.52g Net Carbs, and 18.26g Protein.

Bolognese Zoodle Bake

Ingredients

Bolognese Sauce

1.5 pounds ground beef

1 tablespoon olive oil

½ medium white onion, about 100g or 3.5oz

2-3 cloves of garlic, minced

½ teaspoon thyme

½ teaspoon ground nutmeg

½ teaspoon ground marjoram

2 cups Rao's marinara sauce

2 tablespoons heavy whipping cream

¼ cup chicken bouillon paste

Salt and pepper to taste

Zucchini Noodles

2-3 medium zucchini, about 570g or 20oz

2 tablespoons olive oil

1 cup shredded mozzarella cheese

Salt and pepper to taste

Optional garnish: fresh basil

Instructions

1. Preheat a skillet over medium heat, and set your slow cooker onto "low." Finely dice half of a medium sized white onion while you wait for the skillet to heat up.

2. Add olive oil to the frying pan.

3. Once the oil becomes hot, add the diced onion. Cook until the onions start to become translucent and pick up a bit of color.

4. Stir in the minced garlic cloves.

5. Crumble the ground beef into the pan. Don't worry too much about breaking up the chunks as they cook. Everything is going to fall apart in the slow cooker anyway.

6. Add in ½ a teaspoon of thyme, ½ a teaspoon of nutmeg, ½ a teaspoon of marjoram, and black pepper to taste.

7. Mix everything together and allow the beef to cook until it has mostly browned.

8. Mix in 2 cups of Rao's basil tomato marinara sauce.

9. Stir in the 2 tablespoons of heavy whipping cream.

10. Finish the sauce by mixing in ¼ of a cup of chicken bouillon.

11. Turn the heat off and allow the sauce to rest for about 10 minutes before transferring it into the preheated slow cooker. Be careful not to pour hot sauce into cold stoneware. I've cracked them before!

12. Cover the slow cooker and allow the sauce to simmer for 8 hours. Stir occasionally to prevent burning. When the sauce is ready it will take on a deep color and the house will smell like lasagne. After the sauce has finished cooking you can season with additional salt if needed.

13. Preheat your oven to 350° F.

14. Set up a vegetable spiralizer. Use it to process the zucchini into noodles, and place the noodles in a casserole dish. Break apart the longer strands so that none of them are too long.

15. Add 2 tablespoons of olive oil to the noodles. Season to taste and then mix together.

16. Spread your bolognese sauce over the top of the zucchini.

17. Top the casserole with 1 cup of shredded mozzarella cheese.

18. If baking right after cooking the bolognese sauce, then you will only need to heat the casserole in the oven for 15-20 minutes. If you've made the sauce ahead of time and it's been chilled in the refrigerator then you will need to bake for 30-35 minutes.

19. Garnish with fresh basil if desired.

This makes a total of 6 servings Bolognese Zoodle Bake. Each serving comes out to be 402 Calories, 28.7g Fats, 6g Net Carbs, and 29g Protein.

Beef Brisket

Ingredients

1½ pounds brisket, flank rib, shoulder roast or stew meat

3 cups chicken stock

1 large onion, chopped

8 cloves garlic, peeled and sliced

8 ounces mushrooms, sliced

8 carrots, sliced ½-inch thick

1 tablespoon garlic powder

1 tablespoon onion powder

½ teaspoon celtic sea salt

Instructions

Place stock, onion, garlic, mushrooms, and carrots in crockpot

Sprinkle with garlic powder, onion powder, and salt

Place meat in center

Turn crockpot on to low and cook for 6-8 hours

Serve

Keto Shepherd's Pie

Serves:8

Ingredients

2 tablespoons olive oil

1 large onion, diced

1 pound turkey or pork bacon, cut into ½-inch slices

2 cups diced carrots

2 cups diced celery

1 pound organic grass fed ground beef

½ teaspoon celtic sea salt

1 teaspoon ground black pepper

½ teaspoon smoked paprika

1 cup chicken broth

2 large heads cauliflower, trimmed, chopped and steamed until very soft

2 tablespoons olive oil

Instructions

Heat olive oil in a very large frying pan

Saute onion for 15 minutes until soft

Add bacon pieces to pan and sauté until cooked, about 10 minutes

Add carrots and celery to pan and sauté in bacon fat for 10 minutes until soft

Add ground beef to pan and sauté until brown, just a few minutes

Season with salt, pepper and smoked paprika

Add chicken broth and cook down broth until 60% evaporated

Place cauliflower in food processor and puree with olive oil until smooth

Pour ground beef mixture into a 9 x 13 inch baking dish

Pour mashed cauliflower over beef mixture

Bake at 350° for 30 minutes

Serve

Desserts

Keto Lemon Custard Tarts with Almond Lavender Crust

Serves 2

For the crust

3 tbsp unsalted butter, melted

3/4 cup almond meal

1/2 tbsp dried lavender flowers (optional)

1 tbsp sugar-free vanilla syrup (like Torani)

For the filling

4 large egg yolks

grated zest of 3 lemons

1/2 cup unsalted butter, melted

1/2 cup freshly squeezed lemon juice

1/4-1/2 cup sugar-free vanilla syrup (depends on your preference for a zing, I use 1/4)

Instructions

Preheat oven to 375 degrees fahrenheit

Take two creme brulee dishes (4.5 inches in diameter x 1.25 inches thick) and grease them (I used ghee)

In a mortar and pestle, grind lavender flowers into a fine dust.

Mix lavender, almond flour, and 3 tbsp melted butter

Press mix into the bottom of the dishes.

Bake for 10 minutes or until the tops begin to brown, then remove from oven and set aside.

In a blender or food processor, blend the egg yolks, lemon zest, lemon juice, sweetener, 1/2 cup melted butter until smooth.

Transfer filling to a small saucepan and cook over medium-low heat, stirring constantly with a spatula until thick like pudding (about 15 minutes).

Pour the filling over the almond-lavender crust in the two dishes.

Cover with plastic wrap and refrigerate overnight.

Enjoy!

Keto Strawberry Shortcake Recipe

Ingredients

2 tbsp almond meal

1/2 tbsp butter

1 cup chopped strawberries

1/2 cup cream

If you use sweetener: 1 tsp sugar free vanilla syrup

Instructions

Add the almond meal and butter to a mug and microwave for 30 seconds.

Mix together and flatten to the bottom of your mug, using the bottom of a spoon so that it resembles a flat crust.

Chop up a cup of strawberries (about 4 large strawberries).

Add to the mug and press down.

Blend your heavy cream (and sweetener if you use it).

Add to the to the mug and refrigerate for at least 30 minutes (the crust needs to cool + become shortbread-like).

Enjoy!

Keto Pound Cake

Ingredients

Pound cake

2 1/2 cups almond flour

½ cup unsalted butter, softened

1 1/2 cups erythritol

8 whole eggs, room temperature

1 1/2 tsp. vanilla extract

1/2 tsp. lemon extract

½ tsp. salt

8 oz. cream cheese

1 1/2 tsp. baking powder

Glaze

¼ cup powdered erythritol

3 Tbsp. heavy whipping cream

½ tsp. vanilla extract

Instructions

1. Preheat oven to 350F. Toss in room temperature butter, softened cream cheese, and erythritol into a mixing bowl.

2. Cream together the butter and erythritol until smooth. Then, add in softened chunks of cream cheese and blend together until smooth.

3. Add in the eggs, lemon extract,and vanilla extract in with the blended ingredients. Blend with a hand mixer until smooth.

4. In a medium sized bowl: mix together the almond flour, baking powder, and salt.

5. Slowly add in the ingredients from the medium sized bowl into the batter. Use a hand blender to blend the clumps until very smooth.

6. Pour batter into a loaf pan. Bake for 60 – 120 minutes at 350F or until smooth in the middle when tested with a toothpick.

7. If creating a glaze: blend together the powdered erythritol, vanilla extract, and heavy whipping cream

until smooth. Wait until the pound cake is fully cooled from the oven before spreading the glaze on top.

This makes a total of 16 servings of pound cake. Each slice comes out to be 255.56 Calories, 22.19g Fats, 3.44g Net Carbs, and 6.81g Protein.

Keto Cookies and Crème Ice Cream

Ingredients

Cookie Crumbs

3/4 cup almond flour

1/4 cup cocoa powder

1/4 tsp. baking soda

1/4 cup erythritol

1/2 tsp. vanilla extract

1 1/2 Tbsp. coconut oil, softened

1 egg, room temperature

Pinch of salt

Ice Cream

2 1/2 cups whipping cream

1 Tbsp. vanilla extract

1/2 cup erythritol

1/2 cup almond milk, unsweetened

Instructions

1. Preheat oven to 300F. Line 9 inch circular cake pan with parchment paper and spray with oil of choice.

2. Sift the almond flour, cocoa powder, baking soda, erythritol, and salt into a medium bowl and then whisk until smooth.

3. Add the vanilla extract and coconut oil and mix until batter forms into fine crumbs.

4. Add the egg and blend until cookie batter begins to stick together and form a ball.

5. Transfer the batter into prepared cake pan and press out batter thinly with your fingers until it evenly covers the bottom of the pan.

6. Place pan in preheated oven and bake for 20 minutes or until center of cookie bounces back when pressed.

7. When finished baking, remove pan from oven and let cool.

8. Once the cookie has cooled, break the cookie into small crumbles.

9. In a large bowl, blend the whipping cream with an electric mixer until stiff peaks form.

10. Add vanilla extract and erythritol, and whip until thoroughly combined.

11. Pour in almond milk and blend mixture until it re-thickens.

12. Transfer cream mixture to ice cream maker and churn until ice cream begins to hold its shape.

13. Gradually pour the cookie crumbles in while the ice cream maker is churning to evenly mix the crumbles into the ice cream.

14. Once all of the cookie crumbles are incorporated, transfer the ice cream into a ½ gallon freezer-safe container and freeze for at least 2 hours before serving.

This makes a total of 10 servings Keto Cookies and Crème Ice Cream. Each serving comes out to be 293 Calories, 28.69g Fats, 3.63g Net Carbs, and 4.59g Protein.

Keto Gingersnap Cookies

Ingredients

2 cups almond flour

¼ cup unsalted butter

1 cup erythritol

1 large egg

1 tsp. vanilla extract

¼ tsp. salt

2 tsp. ground ginger

¼ tsp. ground nutmeg

¼ tsp. ground cloves

½ tsp. ground cinnamon

Instructions

1. Preheat oven to 350F. In a large mixing bowl, mix the dry ingredients together.

2. In a small bowl, mix the wet ingredients of melted unsalted butter, egg, and vanilla extract until well combined.

3. Add the wet ingredients to the dry ingredients. Blend with a hand mixer until combined. The cookie batter will be slightly stiff and crumbly.

4. Use a tablespoon to measure out each cookie. Flatten the top of each cookie with a spatula or just use your fingers.

5. Bake for 10-12 minutes at 350F or until they're lightly browned on top.

This makes a total of 24 servings of Gingersnap Cookies. Each cookie comes out to be 74 Calories, 6.71g Fats, 1.21g Net Carbs, and 2.25g Protein.

Drinks

Green Low Carb Breakfast Smoothie

Ingredients

1.5 cups almond milk

1 oz spinach

50 grams cucumber

50 grams celery

50 grams avocado

1 tbsp coconut oil

10 drops liquid stevia

1 scoop Isopure Protein Powder (about 30 grams)

1 tsp matcha powder (optional)

Instructions

Into a blender or Nutribullet, add your almond milk and spinach. Blend for a second to break down the spinach to make room for the rest of the ingredients.

Add in the rest of your ingredients and blend for about a minute until creamy.

You can add a teaspoon of matcha powder for added benefits and a kick of caffeine. Enjoy!

Low Carb Hot Chocolate

Ingredients

1 cup almond milk (or any nut milk)

1/8 cups heavy cream

1.50 tbsps Sukrin Erythritol

1.50 tbsps cocoa powder

1/8 tsps cinnamon

Instructions

Set a small pot onto a low flame with your almond (or any nut) milk and heavy cream. To make this dairy free - use some coconut cream!

While it's heating up, place the rest of your ingredients into a Nutribullet or small blender.

When your milk mixture is bubbling slightly, take it off the flame and pour the contents into your blender.

Blend for about a minute to get it nice and frothy.

Serve with some shaved chocolate and enjoy!

Fruit Infused Iced Tea

Ingredients

2 cups boiled water

1 tea bag

1 strawberry

1 slice lemon

1 doonk Stevia

1 tbsp apple cider vinegar

ice

Instructions

Set a pot of water to boil. Once it's boiled, pour the water into a mug and begin brewing your tea.

Slice a strawberry into small sections and add it along with a slice of lemon into your tea to brew.

Add ice and Stevia to your glass or travel container.

Pour the brewed tea into the container submerging the fruit. Give it a good shake/stir and make sure it's cold enough!

Optionally, you can add a tablespoon of apple cider vinegar for the health benefits it provides.

Iced Matcha Latte

Ingredients

1 cup unsweetened cashew milk

1 tbsp coconut oil

1 tsp matcha powder

1/8 teaspoon vanilla bean

2 ice cubes

Instructions

Combine all ingredients in a blender or Nutribullet and blend until ice cubes are broken down.

Sprinkle some extra matcha on top or even cocoa powder to garnish!

Keto Protein Shake

Ingredients

1 cup almond milk

1 tbsp cocoa powder

1 tbsp coconut oil

1 tbsp peanut butter

2 tsp erythritol

1 scoop chocolate protein powder

4 ice cubes

Instructions

Invest in a good, low carb protein powder! In these cases, the flavor doesn't matter too much as we're adding a whole bunch of goodies. We used Now Foods Chocolate Protein Powder, which is 0 net carbs per serving.

In a Nutribullet, combine all the dry ingredients and then add your wet ones. You can choose your main liquid here. Whether it's water, cream, coconut/almond/cashew milk, make sure it's low carb. Even in innocent almond milk, some brands pump in a good amount of sugar. Try to buy the unsweetened versions.

Add ice cubes for added thickness and blend for about a minute. Enjoy cold!

Snacks

Kale Chips

Ingredients

0.50 bunch kale

1 tbsp olive oil

1 tbsp Parmesan cheese

0.50 tsps garlic powder

0.50 tsps salt

0.50 tsps crushed red pepper

Instructions

Start by washing and drying your bunch of kale. Make sure to dry them really well between some paper towels. If the kale is too wet with water when going in to the oven, it will steam instead of bake.

Rip into your desired pieces. Stem in or out, your preference.

Pour in your oil of choice; we used olive oil. And add in your seasoning.

Using your hands, gently massage and combine all the ingredients and make sure both sides of every leaf are shiny with oil.

Next, lay and space them out on a cookie sheet. We didn't grease ours as our chips were oily enough.

Throw them into the oven at 350° F. After 8 minutes, check in on them. If they're still soft, keep baking for 2 minute intervals. We ended up baking ours for about 12 minutes.

When they're sufficiently crunchy, take them out and tip them over into a deep bowl. They're ready to snack on! Enjoy!

Bacon-Wrapped Jalapeno Poppers

Ingredients

16 fresh jalapeños

16 strips bacon

4 oz cream cheese

1/4 cup shredded cheddar cheese

1 tsp salt

1 tsp paprika

Instructions

Preheat oven to 350° F

Slice the bacon in half (this will give you 16 half length pieces).

Slice the ends off each jalapeno. Slice each jalapeno in half length-wise. Remove seeds and membranes with a corer or knife. (Caution: use gloves to protect hands)

Mix the cream cheese and cheddar cheese together in a bowl.

Fill each jalapeno half with the cheese mix. (You can either place two halves back together or keep them separate. We prefer separate!)

Wrap each piece in bacon.

Place all bacon-wrapped jalapeno poppers on a baking sheet lined with aluminum foil. Make sure there is a bit of room between each piece. Bake for 20-25 minutes (until bacon is baked and jalapenos are desired spiciness).

Important: Do a taste test with one popper to measure the spiciness. The longer you bake the poppers, the less hot they become.

Add salt, paprika and any other spices to taste. Enjoy!

Salted Almond and Coconut Bark

Ingredients

1/6 cups almonds

1/6 cups unsweetened flaked coconut

33.33 g dark chocolate (see notes)

1/6 cups coconut butter

1/6 tsps almond extract (optional)

3.33 drops liquid stevia (optional)

1/12 tsps sea salt

Instructions

Preheat the oven to 350° F. Spread the almonds and coconut onto a foil-lined baking sheet. Place it in the preheated oven and toast for 5-8 minutes. Stir once or twice to prevent burning. Once everything is toasted, set the baking sheet off to the side to cool.

In a double boiler, melt the dark chocolate and stir in the coconut butter once it has melted a bit. Add in the almond extract and liquid stevia (optional). Mix well and set aside.

Line a baking sheet with parchment or wax paper and pour the chocolate mixture in. Spread it out evenly using the back of a spoon or silicone spatula.

Scatter the toasted almond and coconut flakes over the top and press gently with your hands so that everything is touching the chocolate. Sprinkle lightly with sea salt and let it set in the refrigerator for at least an hour.

Once it has set, slice with a knife or a pizza roller. We opted to break/rip it into shards and enjoy their imperfect shapes!

Dippable Crispy Cheddar Cheese Chips {Keto & Low-Carb}

Ingredients

4 cups cheddar cheese, or mexican blend (depends on your size baking sheet, should form a single layer.)

1/2 tsp sea salt

1/2 tsp onion powder

1/4 tsp garlic powder

1/4 tsp cumin

1/4 tsp paprika

1/4 tsp chili powder

Instructions

Preheat an oven to 400F

Line a large baking sheet with parchment paper, leaving a little extra on the side to make it easy to pull up and out of the pan when you're done.

In a bowl, combine cheese and spices.

Spread out over the baking sheet and form into a rectangle with as straight edges as you can.

Bake in the oven for about 20 minutes, or until visibly crispy.

Remove from oven.

Lift the cheese out of the pan with the sides of the parchment paper and place on a cool countertop. (If your cheese is extra droopy, it needs to be cooked longer.)

After about 1 minute of cooling, you should be able to use a pizza cutter and cut your rectangle of cheese into triangles.

Notes

The cheese will go through a few phases when cooking. At first it will be melty, then it will be bubbly, then a bunch of the moisture will cook off and it will begin to get crispy, which is what you want. Once the whole thing looks crispy, you're in good hands. If they end up being flabby and not stiff, just cook them longer next time. All ovens are different!

Pistachio-Crusted Sundried Tomato Goat Cheese Balls

Ingredients

1 4oz package of sundried tomato goat cheese

1/2 cup de-shelled pistachios

salt to taste

Instructions

Cut your goat cheese into 7 slices and form into balls

Use a mortar and pestle to lightly crush your pistachios (don't grind them, whack 'em)

Add salt to the pistachio mixture to taste

Roll your balls around in the pistachio mixture to cover

Once they're all covered, roll one more time in the leftover pistachio dust

Enjoy!

Conclusion

We hope the info in this book has not only satisfied your needs but has made you feel more optimistic about starting the diet and watching the inches disappear.

If you start to falter after starting this diet, remember that the Keto Diet is a proven method for losing weight and improving your over-all health. Following this diet and reaching ketosis can flood you with energy and well-being, which is definitely worth making a few small sacrifices for.

Good luck from here on out, and feel free to review the information in this book from time-to-time to remind yourself of tips that might aid you.

And most of all, enjoy the prospects of buying a new wardrobe for your new silky frame.